Introduction

Hi and Welcome! I am so glad you're here. We live a crazy and hectic life today, it leaves us feeling a bit disconnected. But there is one thing that can help you to feel connected it would be a Yoga practice. Yoga can help with restoring balance and can also improve your physical health and can relieve stress boy we all could use some help there. Life presents all sorts of challenges, from health problems, mental breakdowns and physical ailments and the list goes on. But through yoga and meditation one can again reconnect with one's true self and experience joy, serenity and inner peace.Yoga can also help you gain strength, balance and flexibility. By developing a yoga practice you'll begin the journey towards completely transforming your life. People of all shapes and sizes and experience levels can do yoga! You can practice and benefit from some versions of yoga.

The main objective in this book is to help make your practice of yoga at home easy so you can make it a habit in your everyday life to help improve your health, mind and body. Who wouldn't want to do that? ! It doesn't matter if you're completely brand new to yoga, and it doesn't matter how much you do with yoga – any small step is going to help you. By developing a yoga practice you'll begin the journey towards completely transforming your life. Anyone can do yoga and anyone can benefit from starting a yoga practice and that includes you! This practice is all about you, so let's explore how yoga can fit into your life. But let's first find out what yoga is.

"Yoga is a union of mind, body, and breath," explains Rebecca Young Riboldi, a yoga instructor at FLYLDN. Combining a series of poses with an emphasis on the breath, it's a workout for both your body and your mind. The origins of this ancient practice date back more than 5,000 years to India. The language used in yoga is Sanskrit—one of the oldest languages in the world. And you'll often hear words like āsana and Savasana during practice.

Modern yoga teachings became widely popular in Western countries by the 1970s.

It was during this time that the health and fitness industry was becoming the latest trend. People were flocking to newly opened gyms, fitness clubs, and recreation centers. Weight lifting and group aerobic exercise classes were coming onto the scene.

Hatha Yoga in its various styles, seemed to fit the mold of health and fitness that attracted people to these health centers. Yoga began to make its way into the local gyms and into stand-alone studios.

At first, yoga may have looked like a trend, but we can clearly see that yoga is something that is here to stay.

"Yoga is an incredibly transformational and constantly evolving practice," says Alana Murrin, yoga teacher at Psycle. "It combines mindful movement with breathing techniques, meditation, and yogic philosophy, to help you reach a state of equilibrium and balance in body and mind." Murrin points out some aspects of yoga will feel easier than others, but those you find most challenging will be your most powerful teachers. Patience and commitment are key when it comes to this practice.

The Benefits of Yoga

A regular routine of yoga can benefit you in many ways.

- **Better posture:** By strengthening and stretching the shoulders, chest, back, and abdominal (the areas affected by sitting all day), yoga poses will help you stand taller, live with an open heart, and help to relieve any discomfort that comes with bad posture from sitting.
- **Toning the body:** The connective tissue and muscle fibers get longer and the added resistance creates tension that helps the body build and maintain a toned appearance. For these reasons, yoga is an excellent way to tone virtually every major muscle group including the booty and abs.:
- **Helps build strength and breathing technique:** Slow movements and deep breathing increase blood flow and warm up muscles, while holding a pose can build strength.
- **Better Sleep:** Research show that a consistent bedtime yoga routine can help you get in the right mindset and prepare your body to fall asleep and stay asleep.
- **Increases energy levels:** Recent studies have shown that certain yoga poses reduce fatigue and increase the hormone cortisol. Low levels of

cortisol can zap your energy, leaving you feeling rundown. Enjoying a regular yoga practice will help you maintain healthy cortisol levels.

- **Aids digestion:** Yoga may help relieve digestive issues by decreasing stress, increasing circulation, and promoting gut motility.
- **Reduces the chance of osteoporosis:** It encourages muscle and bone strength, which has a positive effect on your balance, posture, and stability. Staying active can help to alleviate pain and reduce your risk of bone fractures.
- **Helps with arthritis:** Gentle yoga has been shown to ease some of the discomfort of tender, swollen joints for people with arthritis, according to Johns Hopkins.
- **Promotes resilience:** Calming the body. When we release tension in various muscles throughout our body during a yoga pose, we send a message to our brain that it is ok to relax or surrender.
- **Reduces build-up of stress:** According to the National Institutes of Health, scientific evidence shows that yoga supports stress management, mental health, mindfulness, healthy eating, weight loss and quality sleep.
- **Helps develop love and acceptance of your body:** Yoga teaches you to appreciate your own body as it feels rather than how it looks. In this respect, the discipline of regular practice teaches students how to sense, feel and trust their own

bodies, to open their minds and to acknowledge their souls

- **Allows you to discover a deeper connection with yourself:** Consciously uniting the mind and body through breath and posture, yoga induces a positive feeling and makes us more present-minded, focused, and energized.
- **Gives you greater awareness of emotions:** You may feel increased mental and physical energy, a boost in alertness and enthusiasm, and fewer negative feelings after getting into a routine of practicing yoga.
- **Opportunity to connect with like-mind people:** Participating in yoga classes can ease loneliness and provide an environment for group healing and support. Even during one-on-one sessions loneliness is reduced as one is acknowledged as a unique individual, being listened to and participating in the creation of a personalized yoga plan.
- **Relaxation and healing:** the practice of yoga also improves the body's inherent healing abilities. Many yoga poses are often combined in a yoga class to further boost yoga's healing powers.
- **Helps with back pain:** Yoga is as good as basic stretching for easing pain and improving mobility in people with lower back pain. The American College of Physicians recommends yoga as a first-line treatment for chronic low back pain.

As with many practices there are different forms of yoga for each individual. There are six branches of yoga. Each branch represents a different focus and set of characteristics.

The Six Branches of Yoga

1.**Hatha yoga:** This is the physical and mental branch that aims to prime the body and mind.

2.**Raja yoga:** This branch involves meditation and strict adherence to a series of disciplinary steps known as the eight limbs of yoga.

3.**Karma yoga:** This is a path of service that aims to create a future free from negativity and selfishness.

4.**Bhakti yoga:** This aims to establish the path of devotion, a positive way to channel emotions and cultivate acceptance and tolerance.

5.**Jnana yoga**: This branch of yoga is about wisdom, the path of the scholar, and developing the intellect through study.

6.**Tantra yoga:** This is the pathway of ritual, ceremony, or consummation Yoga is an ancient practice that has changed over time.

Modern yoga focuses on poses designed to stimulate inner peace and physical energy. Ancient yoga did not place as much emphasis on fitness. Instead, it revolved around cultivating mental focus and expanding spiritual energy.

12 Types of Yoga

Modern yoga focuses on exercise, strength, agility, and breathing. It can help boost physical and mental well-being.

There are many styles of yoga. A person should choose a style based on their goals and fitness level.

Types and styles of yoga include:

1.Ashtanga yoga

This type of yoga practice uses ancient yoga teachings. However, it became popular during the 1970s.

Ashtanga applies the same poses and sequences that rapidly link every movement to breath.

2.Bikram yoga

People practice Bikram yoga, also known as hot yoga, in artificially heated rooms at a temperature of nearly 105oF and 40% humidity. It consists of 26 poses and a sequence of two breathing exercises.

3.Hatha yoga

This is a generic term for any type of yoga that teaches physical poses. Hatha classes usually serve as a gentle introduction to the basic poses of yoga.

4.Iyengar yoga

This type of yoga practice focuses on finding the correct alignment in each pose with the help of a range of props, such as blocks, blankets, straps, chairs, and bolsters.

5.Kripalu yoga

This type teaches practitioners to know, accept, and learn from the body. A student of Kripalu yoga learns to find their own level of practice by looking inward.

The classes usually begin with breathing exercises and gentle stretches, followed by a series of individual poses and final relaxation.

6.Kundalini yoga

Kundalini yoga is a system of meditation that aims to release pent-up energy.

A Kundalini yoga class typically begins with chanting and ends with singing. In between, it features asana, pranayama, and meditation that aim to create a specific outcome.

7.Power yoga

In the late 1980s, practitioners developed this active and athletic type of yoga based on the traditional Ashtanga system.

8.Sivananda

This system uses a five point philosophy as its foundation.

This philosophy maintains that proper breathing, relaxation, diet, exercise, and positive thinking work together to create a healthy yogic lifestyle.

People practicing Sivananda use 12 basic asanas, which they precede with Sun Salutations and follow with Savasana.

9.Viniyoga

Viniyoga focuses on form over function, breath and adaptation, repetition and holding, and the art and science of sequencing.

10.Yin yoga

Yin yoga places its focus on holding passive poses for long periods of time. This style of yoga targets deep tissues, ligaments, joints, bones, and fascia.

11. Prenatal yoga Prenatal yoga uses poses that practitioners have created with pregnant people in mind. This yoga style can help people get back into shape after giving birth, and support health during pregnancy.

12.Restorative yoga This is a relaxing method of yoga. A person spends a restorative yoga class in four or five simple poses, using props such as blankets and bolsters to sink into deep relaxation without exerting any effort when holding the pose.

Preparing for Yoga

Preparing for yoga requires dedication, time and commitment. It is important to prioritize it into your schedule. Here are some tips to help you get started.

1. Create a comfortable spot for your yoga practice. It is important to have the same space when practicing yoga.
2. Get your yoga accessories. Although you don't need equipment to practice yoga. There are some tools that will help. These tools can be used for asana and meditation along with your yoga practice and they are: yoga mat, yoga blocks, yoga strap, blanket music, incense, oils,

pre recorded meditation music, comfortable clothing.

3. Stay safe, prevent injury. Practice is a quiet, secluded place with comfortable clothes you can easily move in that is not too loose.
4. Choose your yoga style / routine. …
5. Always relax with Savasana. exercise has a profound effect on the body. Your heart beats faster, your body sweats, and your lungs breathe more heavily. So Savasana is a meditation practice that also helps the organs return to regular functioning after exercising, thus aiding recovery.
6. Practice yoga regularly. …Wherever you begin, whether in a local yoga studio or with an online yoga video, there are a few basics to start with.
7. Start with postures, or yoga *asanas*, such as downward-facing dog, child's pose, and *savasana*.
8. In each pose, focus on pressing your hands or feet into the floor, lengthening your spine, and relaxing your hips. If you keep this in mind as you practice, you will be working with each pose exactly as even the most devoted practitioners do.
9. Enjoy your practice! …

So get on your mat, practice and start living better!

First is to learn how to breathe when you start to do yoga or any other kind of exercise.

Concentrate on Breathing

Yoga uses a technique of controlling breathing, or pranayama, which is just as important as the poses you adopt. There are many types of breathing used during yoga; for a complete guide to pranayama consult http://www.yogajournal.com/category/poses/types/pranayama/. The basic three types you will need are:[34]

1. Quiet breathing (natural without effort) – It is typically used during the ending period of relaxation and meditation.
2. Deep breathing (long, deep breaths) - Yoga that focuses on relaxation, or during which the poses are held for a long time, often emphasizes deep breathing.
3. Fast breathing (a deliberate increase in breathing rate) - More exercise-focused yoga that moves quickly from poses to pose often incorporates more fast breathing.

Wherever you begin, whether in a local yoga studio or with an online yoga video, there are a few basics to start with.

Start with postures, or yoga *asanas*, such as downward-facing dog, child's pose, and *savasana*.

In each pose, focus on pressing your hands or feet into the floor, lengthening your spine, and relaxing your hips. If you keep this in mind as you practice, you will be working with each pose exactly as even the most devoted practitioners do. What are the basic yoga steps?

7 Basic Yoga Poses

Mountain Pose (Tadasana) Mountain Pose acts as the foundation for other poses. Mentally, it tests your focus and concentration. On a physical level, it improves your posture, strengthens your thighs, knees, and ankles, firms your abdomen and buttocks, relieves sciatica, and reduces flat feet. Stand with the feel parallel, a few inches apart. (Alternately you may stand with the bases of your big toes touching, heels slightly apart.

Rotate both thighs inward and engage your quads, drawing them upward throughout the pose.

Lift and spread your toes and the balls of your feet, then lay them softly back down on the floor. Rock gently back and forth and side to side. Gradually reduce this swaying to a standstill, with your weight balanced evenly across your feet. Feel the energy draw from your feet up through your core.

Without pushing your lower front ribs forward, lift the top of your sternum straight toward the ceiling. Widen your collarbones. Allow your shoulder blades to draw toward each other and down the back, away from the ears.

Let your arms relax beside your torso, palms facing in or forward.

Balance the crown of your head directly over the center of your pelvis, with the underside of your chin parallel to the floor, throat soft, and tongue wide and flat on the floor of your mouth. Soften your eyes. Breathe.

Child's Pose (Balasana)

Child's Pose is a gentle stretch for the back, hips, thighs, and ankles. It can help relieve back pain.

Learning to use this pose wisely is the part of your developing practice where you listen to your body's inner voice and do what it tells you. Your body will tell you when to rest. It might need different things on different days. Keeping your ear finely tuned to the messages your body is sending you and respectfully responding to them is the greatest lesson that a child's pose has to offer. You will come to know when to use Child's Pose during your yoga practice.

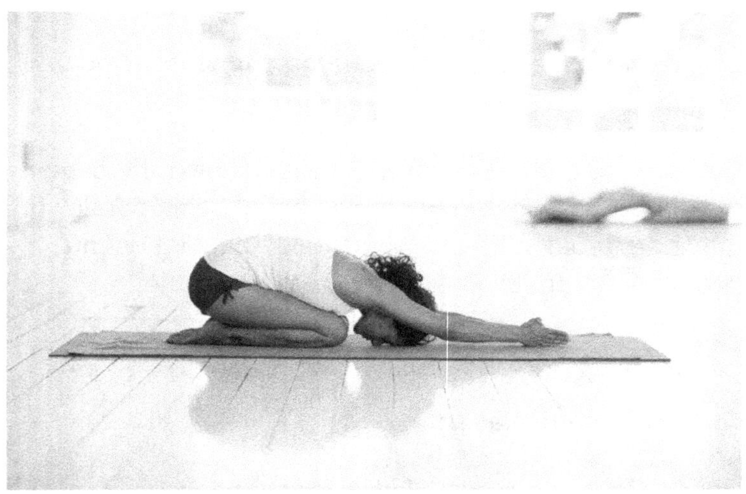

Step-by-Step Instructions

1. Come to your hands and knees on the yoga mat.
2. Spread your knees as wide as your mat, keeping the tops of your feet on the floor with the big toes touching.
3. Bring your belly to rest between your thighs and root your forehead to the floor. Relax the shoulders, jaw, and eyes. If it is not comfortable to place the forehead on the floor, rest it on a block or two stacked fists. There is an energy point at the center of the forehead in between the eyebrows that stimulates the vagus nerve and supports a "rest and digest" response. Finding a comfortable place for the forehead is key to gaining this soothing benefit.
4. There are several possible arm variations. You can stretch your arms in front of you with the palms toward the floor or bring your arms back alongside your thighs with the palms facing upwards. These are the most common variations. But you can also stretch the arms forward with palms facing up for a shoulder release or try bending the elbows so that the palms touch and rest the thumbs at the back of the neck. In this position inch the elbows forward.
5. Do whichever feel more comfortable for you. If you've been doing a lot of shoulder work, the second option feels nice.

6. Stay as long as you like, eventually reconnecting with the steady inhales and exhales of your breath.

Cat/Cow Pose (Marjaryasana to Bitilasana)

Keep your hands shoulder-width apart and your knees directly below your hips. Inhale deeply while curving your lower back and bringing your head up, tilting your pelvis up like a "cow." Exhale deeply and bring your abdomen in, arching your spine and bringing your head and pelvis down like a "cat." Repeat several times. What is a cat cow pose good for?

Cat cow pose increases the flexibility of the neck, shoulders and spine. The movement also stretches the muscles of the hips, back, abdomen and chest. Strengthens your spine. During this stretch, it activates the tailbone and releases tension of the neck and upper back.

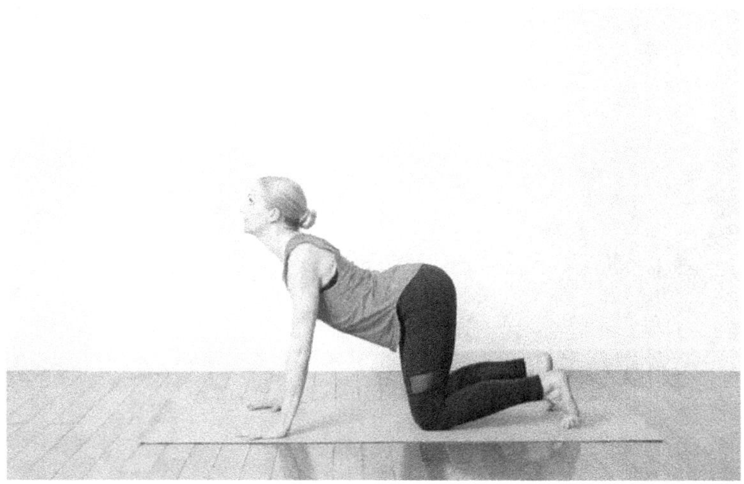

Inhale and Arch for Cow Pose

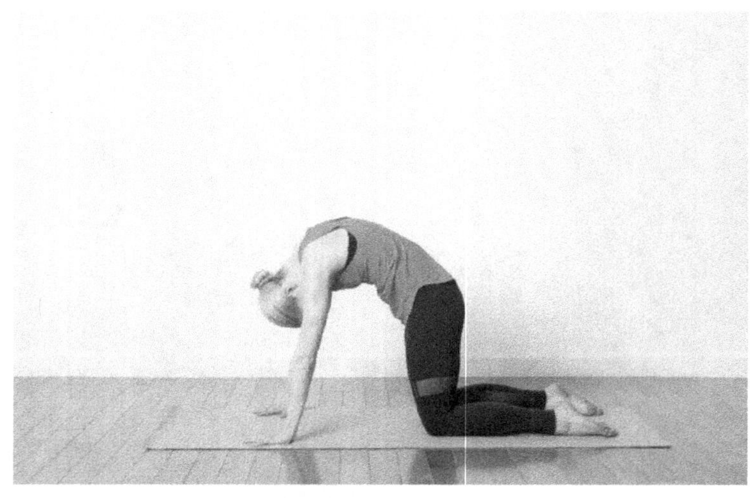

Exhale and Round for Cat Pose

Downward-Facing Dog (Adho Mukha Svanansana)
What is downward-facing dog Good For?

In downward dog, your head is lower than your heart, so it has the benefits of inversions and improves the blood flow through your body. Downward dog stretches and helps to relieve tension from the neck and back. The flow of blood to the brain helps to relieve headaches, mental fogginess, and mild depression.

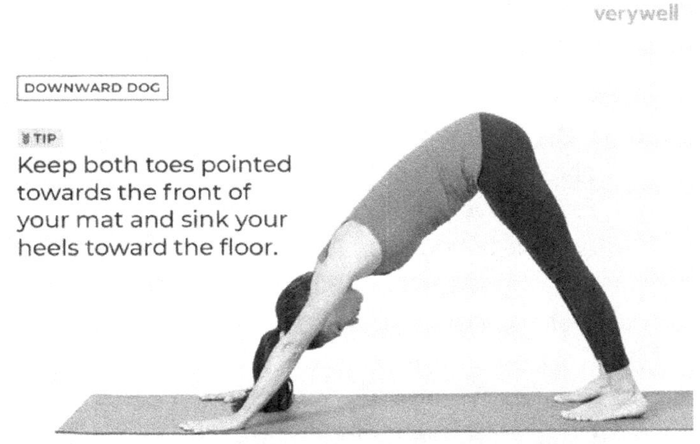

Step-by-Step Instructions

You can do this pose anywhere you can lay out a yoga mat.

1. Come to your hands and knees with your wrists underneath the shoulders and your knees underneath the hips.
2. Curl your toes under and push back through your hands to lift your hips and straighten your legs.
3. Spread your fingers and ground down from the forearms into the fingertips.
4. Outwardly rotate your upper arms to broaden the collarbones.
5. Let your head hang and move your shoulder blades away from your ears towards your hips.
6. Engage your quadriceps strongly to take the burden of your body's weight off your arms. This action goes a long way toward making this a resting pose.
7. Rotate your thighs inward, keep your tail high, and sink your heels towards the floor.
8. Check that the distance between your hands and feet is correct by coming forward to a plank position. The distance between the hands and feet should be the same in these two poses. Do not step the feet toward the hands in Down Dog in order to get the heels to the floor.
9. Exhale and bend your knees to release and come back to your hands and knees.

10. **Warrior I (Virabhadrasana I)** Warrior 1 stretches your chest, lungs, shoulders, neck, belly and groin. It also strengthens your shoulders, arms, and back muscles, as well as your calves, ankles, and thighs.

From <u>Adho Mukha Svanasana (Downward-Facing Dog Pose)</u>, step your right foot forward so your toes are in line with your fingertips, and shift your foot slightly to the right.

1. Bend your front knee 90 degrees. Your thigh should be approximately parallel to the floor, your knee stacked over your ankle, and your right outer hip pinned back.
2. Pivot your left heel to the floor so your foot forms a 45-degree angle to the side of the mat. Align your left heel with your right heel, or place the feet slightly wider for more stability.
3. Press your left thighbone back so your left knee is straight.
4. As you inhale, raise your torso and reach up with the arms, hands shoulder-distance apart and palms facing each other. Allow your sho

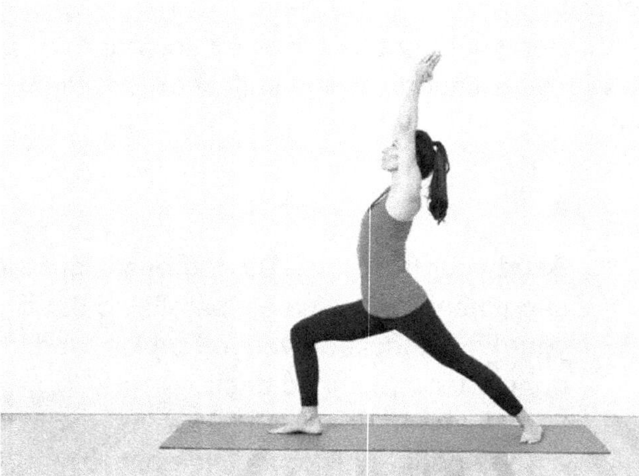

ulder blades to open out and up, away from your spine and toward your outer armpits. Rotate your biceps back, and firm your triceps into your midline. You may bring your palms together and look up at your thumbs.

5. Keep pressing your left femur back while releasing your tailbone toward the floor. Draw your lower belly back and up away from your right thigh.
6. Hold for 5–10 breaths.
7. Release your hands to the floor, step back to Downward-Facing Dog, and repeat on the other side.

Warrior II (Virabhadrasana II)

Benefits of Warrior 2 pose

1.Opens the hips and shoulders.

2.Stretches the inner thighs, groin, and chest.

3.Strengthens the legs, abs, and arms.

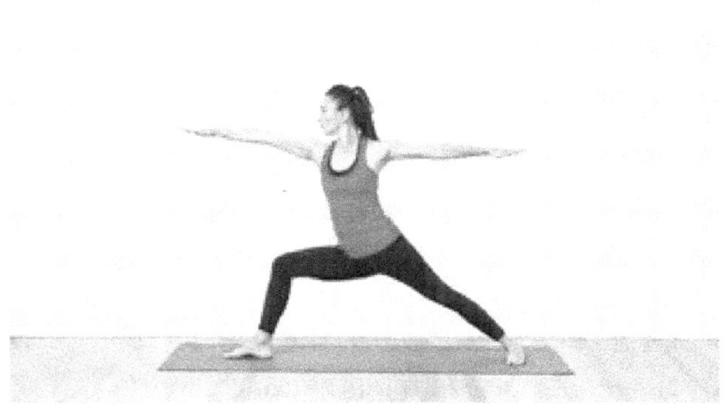

Warrior 2 Pose is a standing strength pose meant to energize the body and mind, increasing concentration and stamina. The posture strengthens the legs as it opens up the chest and hips.

Step by step

1.To come into Warrior 2 pose, start in <u>Tadasana /
Mountain pose</u> at the front of your mat and take a big
step back with your left leg, toes pointing slightly in.

2.Press the four corners of your feet down, and firm your
legs up.

3.As you inhale, raise your arms parallel to the floor,
keeping your shoulders down and your neck long.

4.As you exhale, bend your right knee, keeping your
knee over your ankle. If needed, slightly adjust the
position of your feet and legs to find stability in the pose.

5.Roll the top of your thigh down towards the floor on
the right. Press down through your big toe to balance
that action.

6.Press the top of your left thigh back, and ground the
outside of your left foot into the floor.

7.Draw your lower abdomen in and up and lengthen
your spine. Extend through your collarbones and

fingertips. Bring your chin slightly in and back to align your neck with your spine. Look over your right hand.

8.Stay in this pose for 5 breaths. To come out of the pose press into your feet and straighten your legs as you inhale. Switch the orientation of your feet and repeat on the other side.

Corpse Pose (Shavasana) What are the benefits of corpse pose?

Savasana (Corpse Pose) is much more than a moment's rest at the end of a yoga class.

Calms the central nervous system, aiding the digestive and immune systems.

Calms the mind and reduces stress.

Reduces headache, fatigue and anxiety.

Helps lower blood pressure.

Promotes spiritual awakening and awareness of higher consciousness.

How to do the Corpse Pose:

1. Lie on your back with your legs straight and arms at your sides. Rest your hands about six inches away from your body with your palms up. Let your feet drop open. Close your eyes. You may want to cover your body with a <u>blanket</u>.
2. Let your breath occur naturally.
3. Allow your body to feel heavy on the ground.
4. Working from the soles of your feet up to the crown of your head, consciously release every body part, organ, and cell.
5. Relax your face. Let your eyes drop deep into their sockets. Invite peace and silence into your mind, body, and soul.
6. Stay in Savasana for five minutes for every 30 minutes of your practice.
7. To exit the pose, first begin to deepen your breath. Bringing gentle movement and awareness back to your body, wiggling your fingers and toes. Roll to your right side and rest there for a moment. With an inhalation, gently press yourself into a comfortable seated position. Let your head be the last thing to come into place. Carry the peace and stillness of Savasana with you throughout the rest of your day.

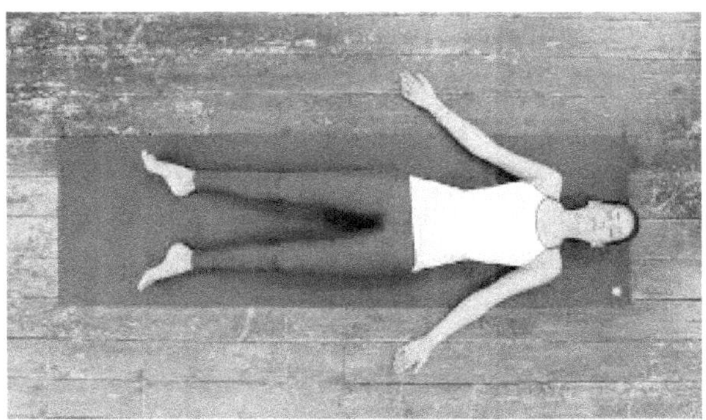

Meditation

"One thing that has helped me get more out of my yoga practice is an interest in understanding and practicing meditation," Young Riboldi says. "There are many apps that make it accessible these days, and it is really a great skill to practice that is extremely complementary to a yoga practice." Yoga's incorporation of meditation and breathing can help improve a person's mental well-being.

Before your first mouthful of coffee in the morning, take a few moments to breathe deeply in through your nose and out through your mouth. "As you get more used to breath work and meditation, you'll find it appears more in your life unconsciously—whether that's a walk around the park, or five minutes of peace when you wake up, that all counts and will have great mindful benefits," explains Chatty Dobson, yoga teacher and owner of <u>FLEX Chelsea</u>.

The square breathing method is a great technique to get you started:

· Close your eyes and visualize a square in your mind's eye

· As you breathe follow the sides of the square in your mind

· Breathe in for a count of 4

· Hold for a count of 4

· Breathe out for a count of 4

· Pause for a count of 4

This is the basics of Yoga and a great way to start your yoga practice for a better you! Learning Yoga, breathing techniques and meditation has helped me and will help you to reconnect and restore your sanity when it comes to dealing with everyday situations.

Summary

  Yoga is an ancient practice that has changed over time.

Modern yoga focuses on poses designed to stimulate inner peace and physical energy. Ancient yoga did not place as much emphasis on fitness. Instead, it revolved around cultivating mental focus and expanding spiritual energy but in today's practice of yoga it also focuses on fitness.

There are many different types of yoga available. The style a person chooses will depend on their expectations and level of physical agility.

People with certain health conditions, such as sciatica, should approach yoga slowly and with caution.

Yoga can help support a balanced, active lifestyle.

Thank you for reading this book. If you have found this book helpful in your journey to learn Yoga. I'd be very appreciative if you would leave a favorable review for this book on Amazon! Thank you. Enjoy your new way of life!

Conclusion

There you have it! Step by Step instructions on how to start a Yoga practice. I hope you really enjoyed reading this book. I know it will help you in so many ways.

If you found this book helpful, Please leave a favorable review for the book on Amazon. I would greatly appreciate it.

"Life isn't about finding yourself, it's about creating yourself." -George Bernard Shaw

Go out and create the best version of you!

Resources

Mike, G. (2021, November 8). *History of Yoga. Origin of yoga. Timeline.* History of Yoga. Origin of Yoga. Timeline. Retrieved August 4, 2022, from http://yogigo.com/history-of-yoga-timeline/

9 Benefits of Yoga. (n.d.). John Hopkins. Retrieved August 5, 2022, from https://dailyburn.com/life/fitness/ease-lower-back-pain-yoga-poses/g/health/wellness-and-prevention/9-benefits-of-yoga

Sullivan, C. (2021, April 13). *Medical News Today.* Medicalnewstoday. Retrieved August 5, 2022, from https://www.medicalnewstoday.com/articles/286745#philosophy

Marturana Winderl, C.P.T., A. (2018, August 28). *12 must- know yoga poses for beginners*. 12 Must-Know Yoga Poses for Beginners. Retrieved August 5, 2022, from https://www.self.com/gallery/must-know-yoga-poses-for-beginnersYu, C.

(2021, November 2). *The Beginner's Guide to Every Type of Yoga Out There*. Daily Burn Life. Retrieved August 5, 2022, from https://dailyburn.com/life/fitness/yoga-for-beginners-kundalini-yin-bikram/

McGinley, C. (2021, November 18). *Yoga for beginners—how to get into yoga whatever your age or fitness level*. Yoga for Beginners—How to Get into Yoga Whatever Your Age or Fitness Level. Retrieved August 5, 2022, from https://www.womanandhome.com/us/health-wellbeing/fitness/yoga-for-beginners/

Yu, C. (2017, April 24). *8 Yoga Poses to Help Ease Lower Back Pain*. Daily Burn Life. Retrieved August 5, 2022, from https://dailyburn.com/life/fitness/ease-lower-back-pain-yoga-poses/

Oyang, E. (2022, April 5). *How to preform Yoga*. WikiHow. Retrieved August 5, 2022, from https://www.wikihow.com/Perform-Yoga

Yoga Poses A-Z. (n.d.). Yoga Journal. Retrieved August 5, 2022, from https://www.yogajournal.com/pose-finder/pose-finder/

Kraftsow, G. (n.d.). *What is Viniyoga*. American Viniyoga Institute. Retrieved August 5, 2022, from https://viniyoga.com

Warrior 2 Pose. (n.d.). Ekhartyoga. Retrieved August 5, 2022, from https://ekhartyoga.com

Flex Chelea. (n.d.). Flex Chelsea. Retrieved August 5, 2022, from https://flexchelsea.com